The Ultimate Spirituality BOX SET

LEARN TO MASTER CHAKRAS, ZEN, REIKI AND KUNDALINI

4 in 1 Master Class BOX SET

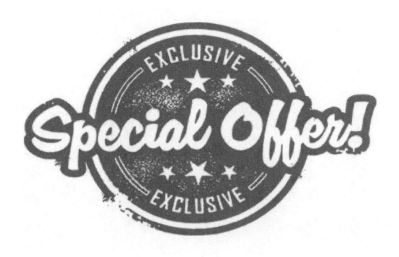

Copyright © 2015

Table of Contents

Book # 1

Chakras

The Ultimate Guide to Mastering Chakras for Beginners in 30 Minutes or Less!

Introduction

I want to thank you and congratulate you for downloading the book, "Chakras - The Ultimate Guide to Mastering Chakras For Beginners in 30 Minutes or Less!"

This book contains proven steps and strategies for mastering Chakras and their activation.

If you take the time to read this book fully and apply the information held within, this book will help you to live a balanced life with a greater control on your behavior, and reach a level of spirituality which will help you in establishing a connection with your soul.

Thanks again for downloading this book, I hope you enjoy it!

Chapter 1: Chakra: An Introduction

The word chakra has arisen from Sanskrit language, and it was originally called "cakra". Cakra was used to refer to a wheel or a circle. Later on, the term Chakra was developed to refer to spiritual power centers in a person. There are seven types of spiritual powers in Hindu religion and one of them is chakra. This term is used in yoga and also in Hindu culture where it is used to refer to the energy nodes of the body. It is believed that there are power points in the human body which are not exactly in the human's physical form but exist in the subtle sense. These energy points meet at certain places in the subtle body to form channels of energy. These channels of energy are known as Nadiis. Nadiis help in providing the energy for the body that is vital for its movement. This, in the end, helps in giving motion to life and making it full of energy. It is important to note that numerous chakras have been reported in the subtle body, but only seven of them are considered to be important. In terms of yoga, chakras are known as whirlpool and sometimes vortex.

The word Chakra also has its roots in Greek, Lithuanian, Proto-Indo-European and Tocharian terms, all of which refer to a circle or a wheel. Some cultures and texts describe it in the form of the circle of life and the birth and death process. Many theorists have stated that this word has numerous definitions and different explanations. It has been used by different religions and regions, each in their own way. There is no specific type of chakra. Its types merge from the explanation it gets from different sources. In the Sanskrit context, this term is used to mean one or all of the following things.

1. It refers to Shakti or energy. The circle demonstrates the motion of Shakti or its rotation in life.

2. It refers to people in life and the circle they form around a person.

3. It also refers to the diagrams which are mystic in nature.

4. Importantly, it denotes the meaning of nerve system in the body.

However, the Buddhist religion interprets this term differently. It states that the cycle refers to the stages of rebirth which are six in number.

According to David Gordon, there is no particular form for chakras and there is no one system. Chakras develop in accordance with the person performing them. Every teacher would have his preferred chakras or he would pick those chakras that are up to his requirements from a pool of chakras. Hence, every expert considers physical form of the body that pleases his thoughts about chakras. Among the common features of chakras are the following.

- They are used to refer to some part of the human body.

- They are used to refer to the breathing channel and air.

- Usually, they are thought to be located in the center or near the center of the breathing channel.

- There are crossings of channels which give it a spoke like structure or are referred to as the petals of the circle.

- The central channel is crossed by two other channels.

- Different colors are used to draw them or differentiate between them.

This concept was largely developed in the Indian societies and it reached the western societies gradually and slowly. It was in 1927 that the term was properly introduced to the west by John Woodroffe. John had basically translated two important books on chakras called 'sat cakra nirupana' and 'padaka pancaka'. The translation was given a name called 'The Serpent Power'. This book became the gateway for other western writers to present their understanding of the Chakras.

The Modern World Understanding of Chakras

In the modern world, chakras are referred to as the filters in the body which process every type of information and make a database in the body cells. The position of chakras in the body is defined as an aligned pattern starting from the end of spinal cord and going to the top until they reach the head. They move in an ascending order from the lower point of the spine to the head. Now in the modern studies of chakras, a color is ascribed to a certain type of chakra which helps in differentiating it from the other chakras. Chakras have been reported to stand for particular physiological features such as the consciousness of a person. They denote particular important features of a person's body or physiological structure. Every chakra is said to have its own spokes or petals emerging out of it. Hence, this gives it a flower like pattern or a wheel form.

Chakras are known for providing energy to the body and for helping in the interaction of emotions and physical structure of a person. Some experts call it pivot of the body as they refer to the energy center of the body. Chakras help in keeping the body in balance as they tend to move or spin and bring energy from physical activities and emotions to the center of the body. The concept revolves around the belief that the soul of a person is immortal and the body is not. Hence, chakras tend to bring balance between the immortal and the mortal form of life within the human body.

It is said that the chakra concerned with consciousness (called Sahasrara) is located at the top most level of spirituality. The chakra linked with matter is called Muladhara and is at the bottom of the spirituality level. Muladhara is concerned with condensed form of consciousness. Most of the time, it is reported, people performing chakras have to give up on their worldly temptations such as some kind of food.

Chapter 2: Types of Chakras

Though it is said that every expert or teacher comes up with his favorite chakra, there are seven basic types of chakras. These seven basic ones are the central positions of energy in our body. If every transfer or transmission is blocked in any one of these seven chakras, a person can become sick or ill. Hence, knowing the location and the features of each chakra is important.

- **Root Chakra**

  As the name suggests, this chakra represents our base and it enables us to feel stable. Root chakra tells about a person's foundation. It is located near the tailbone which is around the spine's base. It controls emotional areas which revolve around money, basic needs of life and financial issues.

- **Sacral Chakra**

  This chakra is concerned with the feelings of adventure and new experience. It helps in preparing a person for accepting or rejecting a new experience. It builds connections. This chakra is located near the navel in the lower part of the abdomen. It is reported that it is 2 inches from the skin and downwards from the navel point. It controls emotional areas of sexual feelings, pleasure, happiness and well-being.

- **Solar Plexus Chakra**

  This chakra is concerned with the ability of a person to control his life and be confident about it. It is located in the abdomen near the stomach. It controls emotions of esteem, respect, confidence and self-worth.

- **Heart Chakra**

  This chakra is concerned with the feelings of love. It determines the person's ability to love others. It is located near the heart in the chest of a person. It controls emotions of love, peace of soul and happiness.

- **Throat Chakra**

  This chakra is located in the throat of a person and is concerned with the communication aspect of a person. It controls the emotions of talking with others, feeling surrounded, expressing one's self and telling the truth.

- **Third Eye Chakra**

  This chakra is about the ability of a person to know all aspects of a scenario analyze the bigger picture and stay focused. Sometimes, this chakra is referred to as the brow chakra since it is located near the brows. Its location is said to be between the two brows on the forehead. It controls the areas of intellectual thinking, decision making power, wisdom and intuition.

- **Crown Chakra**

  This chakra is known as the highest level chakra in the human body. It enables a person to get full connection with his soul and it leads to spirituality in the full form. It is located at the top of the head and it controls areas of feeling blissful, connecting heart with soul and realizing inner beauty along with the physical one.

As you can see, each chakra has its distinct role. They start from the base of spine and move to the top of the head, and each chakra's location is relevant to its role.

Chapter 3: How to Activate your Chakras

Since chakras are about your energy system, you need to know how well your energy is or how healthy your system is. For this purpose, a number of methods exist. It is very important to understand the system of your body before doing something that would hinder your system's ability. If the system is not worked on properly, it will lead to poor result or at times and it can be hazardous for the body.

The most important thing here is to activate the energy system of your body and locate your chakras. Chakras can be activated by vibrational cleansing process through the use of things like choming essences. These help in the detoxification of your system and they give more energy to your physical structure. As mentioned above, if there is any blockage in the chakras, it can result in any kind of illness. Vibrational cleansing results in removing blockages and helps in repairing your system. However, it is important to note that if there are any damages in your system, they will not be healed easily.

Another way of activating chakras is to use white sage for smudging. This process helps in cleansing negative energy from your body. To do this, you have to burn a white sage while keeping the room closed so that the smoke from the burning sage fills the room. It is said that this process helps in removing negative energy from your house as well.

A third way of activating your chakras is to ask an expert to run their hands down your chakra spots in a specialized manner called auric brushing. Usually, professionals use special gems or stones for this purpose as they believe that certain gems have the power to heal your body spiritually. However, care must be taken in choosing the gem or stone as only specific types of stones can help. Choosing the wrong gem can result in damaging the chakras and this can aggravate the blockage of your energy paths.

The fourth way is to concentrate on your diet and choose a healthy one. Drinking lots of water helps too. Getting the right amount of sleep and sleeping properly at night also helps. Sleep prevents a person from stress and relieving stress results in opening the energy channels of the body.

The fifth method is to breathe a good amount of air. Taking deep breaths results in the provision of energy to the body and it helps in overcoming the blockages.

The sixth way of activating chakras is to take interest in nature and try to interact with your environment. Nature has a blend of different colors which help in healing your soul. There are certain colors that help in giving energy to your body or opening the energy channels. These colors vary from person to person. This is because colors produce different vibrations in different people. It is said that the color green has healing powers and that it is good for the soul. This is why going out and observing nature helps in healing your soul and helps you to feel better. A good practice is to go out for a walk, take deep breaths and think that you are breathing in the colors around you. This helps in feeling energized to a large extent.

Another way of activating chakras is to use particular types of music or sounds. Sound has the power to bring vibrations to your body and it can help in opening energy channels.

The eighth method of chakra activation is to stimulate your intellectual thoughts. This helps in increasing brain activity which is necessary for having a healthy body. If your brain is functioning properly, you will be able to control your chakras with your mind. It helps in activating your chakras and removing any blockages you might have. Another reason for focusing on the brain is because one of your chakras rests in your brain. It is also the highest level chakra of your body. Hence, improving brain activity helps in improving the overall chakra system and the energy level of a person.

In addition to this, meditation helps a lot in bringing peace to the inner self. It helps in removing negative energy from the body and communicating with your inner power zone. Meditation brings you to the point where you separate yourself from the world and think about your inner needs only. This means that you focus on your soul rather than your bodily needs. Hence, it helps you to find peace with yourself and to let your mind connects with your soul. This leads to the activation of your chakras when you are relaxed.

The next rule is to have faith in yourself, be happy with what you get and love the original form of yourself. This brings peace inside your mind and body and helps you to connect with your soul. When a person starts loving himself, his worldly and mortal desires start vanishing. It helps him in focusing on his soul and immortal form, which leads to energy channels' activation. Another thing is to love those around you. This reduces negative feelings of jealousy and helps in bring harmony with the soul. It is a proven scientific fact that when a person gets mad at someone, his body produces harmful chemicals which ultimately result in negative energy. On the other hand, when a person smiles or loves someone, his body gives him positive strength.

It is important to note that if a person is not able to take control of his emotions, he will not be able to take control of his energy. It is vital to own your emotions first and be bold enough to express them. When emotions are kept inside, they tend to become stronger and they turn into a constant bother. This leads to an uneasy feeling which hinders proper sleep, disrupts the sleep cycle and wastes a lot of energy. This is, hence, a blockage of the energy channels and the chakras. Chakras have a close relationship with emotions, and if emotions are suppressed, they damage the chakras along with the soul. To bring harmony to your mind and soul, it is better to express yourself. For example, if a person is mad at someone for a long time and does not express his anger to him or tells that person that his habit is bothering him, he will waste a lot of his time and energy in ill thoughts about the other person. Ultimately, this will damage his chakras.

In addition to this, if a person brings a sense of creativity in his life, his energy channels are not blocked. Creativity sharpens the brain and helps in promoting the balance between soul and body. It leads to a better function performed by the chakras. It is important to note that creativity can be demonstrated in anything as long as it interests you and gives you an exploration bug.

A great way to save your energy channel from blockage is to act in a moral and ethical way. When a person does unethical things or performs activities that involve cheating, lying and deceiving, his energy channels are diverted to the negative side. It damages the balance between his soul and body and ultimately it blocks his energy paths. The energy system of a person is largely dependent on his efforts to act with as much integrity as possible.

Chapter 4: Significance of the Seven Chakras

Starting from the top most chakra, this chapter will enlighten about the features, attributes and the underlying qualities of each chakra.

Crown Chakra

This chakra is the top most level of energy and is at the top of our head. It is known as Sahasrara in Sanskrit and its color is violet. The symbol used to present this chakra is a lotus flower with thousands of petals. The spiritual significance of this chakra is that it represents Shiva or consciousness. Since it is at the top, it shows the unification of all colors and can be taken as the prism of the body. This chakra denotes the attributes of intelligence and Divine mercy in the form of wisdom. It is associated with the pineal gland in the body and it gives energy to this gland for efficient function. Its region is usually described as the upper part of brain towards the right eye. The stone or gem associated with this chakra is pearl which shows purification and quality. This chakra is connected with the motion of planet Pluto, and the person who possesses this chakra is known as an ego maniac or the leader. This chakra denotes that the possessor has intelligence and enlightenment of a number of things. Most importantly, this chakra is known to be the place where the connecting point with the spirit exists. Crown chakra has the responsibility of integrating all the activities performed by the other chakras. It controls the lower level chakras and it is paired with level one or the root chakra. It is said that the lower level chakras once controlled help in reaching a level of spirituality.

Third Eye Chakra

This is the sixth level chakra which is also known as the Ajna. This chakra is located on the forehead near the brows or between the two eyes. It is denoted by indigo color and it has its origins in a seed or Aum. The symbol used to represent this chakra is a triangle which descends in a circle. This chakra is a representation of light or intuition. Reaching this chakra involves the skills of mastering one's own self. It leads to intuition and wisdom along with polishing of the imaginative ability. The organ it influences is the pituitary gland, but it has its impact on a number of other body parts such as the brain, eyes, ears, nose and the spinal cord. The stone it is associated with is diamond and its planet is sun. This shows the power of this chakra as sun is a symbol of illumination. It is also known for triggering the sixth sense in a person and touching the higher states of mind. This chakra connects with the sacral chakra which lies on the second level. Excessive use or activity of this chakra results in an increased analytical and intellectual sense. If this chakra is underactive, it leads to confusion and lack of clarity in thoughts. This chakra is also known for inculcating the qualities of forgiveness and compassion in a person. It makes a person kinder towards the other people and helps in awakening the spirit inside a person. This is why it is named as the third eye chakra; as the third eye is the eye of our soul, the immortal eye.

Throat Chakra

This is the fifth level chakra which is also called Vishuddha in Sanskrit. This lies in the throat region of a person and has light blue color for its representation. The seed of this chakra is Hum and its symbol is a slight modification of the symbol used for the sixth chakra; it's a circle which lies within a triangle which is descending. The location of this chakra shows its function as well as it is used for betterment of speech and communication. It brings creativity, helps in promoting intuitive thoughts and inculcates the desire of speaking and interacting with others. It leads to self-expression and pushes a person to speak truth. It controls the throat area along with the thyroid gland, lungs, digestive track and both arms. It is associated with sapphire as its stone and its motion is linked with the planet of Saturn. The sense linked with this chakra is of hearing and its combination is with level three is called the solar chakra. Excess of this chakra's activity leads to judgmental thoughts about others and can sometimes lead to a hurtful speech for others. Less activity of this chakra results in poor expression of feeling and low level of confidence. This chakra is basically the communication hub of the body. It is responsible for the creativity of a person and helps in making a person realize the need of telling the truth. Sometimes, we feel like someone inside us talks to us and pushes us to tell the truth. That voice is generated by this chakra. Hence, this chakra helps in maintaining relationships with others and connects the world with the soul.

Heart Chakra

The fourth chakra is the heart chakra which is known as the Anahata in Sanskrit. This chakra lies in the center of the human chest and is referred to with the pink or green color. This chakra has a seed of Yum and its symbol is of two triangles, one is ascending and the other is descending, and they are intertwined. This chakra is a representative of air and it gives feelings of love and compassion. A person who is able to activate this chakra is known to possess features of an open heart, balanced emotions and he brings harmony to other people. This chakra is associated with the organs of heart, lungs, liver, and thymus, and it leads to smooth blood circulation. It is represented by ruby as its gem component and its planet is Venus. This chakra helps in improving the sense of touch and it has no other pair among the chakras. It is paired with itself. Excessive activation of this chakra results in an emotional expression which is unfitting for the situation and can also result in poor emotional expression. If this chakra's energy is deficient, it leads to ruthless behavior and the person is devoid of emotions. This chakra, hence, is the center of love and emotions. It is also the central chakra among all the chakras and is therefore considered as a bridge between the higher and lower ones.

Solar Plexus Chakra

This chakra is known as Manipura in Sanskrit and is referred as the 'illustrious gem'. It is characterized by the yellow color and its seed is Ram. The symbol used for this chakra is a triangle with a downward or descending shape. This chakra is characterized by fire since it has solar features. It gives the feelings of power and happiness, and it brings self-esteem. It enables the person to feel motivated and to master his will. It also helps in improving relations with others. The organs that are linked with this chakra include the pancreas, lives, bladder and the stomach. It is characterized by the stone of emerald and its planet is Jupiter. It is linked with the fifth chakra and its excess leads to egotistical thoughts. Its deficiency leads to low self-worth. It is located in the middle of the body and is at the place where most of the energy is centered.

Sacral chakra

This chakra is characterized by the color orange, by the planet of Mercury and it has a seed of Vam. It is known as Swadhistana in Sanskrit and its symbol is of an upward shaped crescent. Its matter is water and it improves relationships, sexuality and the feelings of empathy towards others. Its gem is Amethyst and it controls the sense of taste. It is linked with legs and reproductive organs and its excess leads to addictive feeling. Deficiency of this chakra leads to a shutdown of emotions.

Root Chakra

This chakra is known as the Muladhara and is located at the end of spinal cord. It is characterized by the color red, the planet of mars and the coral gem stone. Its symbol is a square and its matter is earth. It is known to give the feelings of stability and trust. It controls kidneys, spine, bladder and the sense of smell. If it is in excess, it gives the feeling of possessiveness and if deficient, it ends up in lack of stability.

Chapter 5: Chakras and the Types of Energy Channels

Throughout the text, there has been a lot of mention of the energy channels, but what exactly are these channels? This chapter will discuss this in depth.

There are three types of energy channels known as the energy shafts in the body of a person. These shafts start off from the spine in human beings. There is an energy channel at central position known as the Shushumna. The two other channels of energy run parallel to this central one and are named as Pingala and Ida. Pingala is on the right side of Shushumna and Ida is on its left side. In the bigger context, these three energy shafts run parallel to the spine of a person. Now the question arises about how these shafts help in the creation of chakras. The answer is quite simple. Chakras appear at the places where these three types of energy channels meet and start ascending along the spinal cord.

What chakras do is that they collect the Prana or the life force energy. They, then, transform the energy from Prana into other forms and transmit it to other areas of the body. Many of us remain confused about the significance of chakras for our mortal forms. It is usually believed that chakras are only for the spiritual health or for the soul. However, they are equally important for the physical form of a person. They help in the transmission of energy as has been mentioned before. Without chakras, it will not be possible to move energy from one point to another and the existence of the material body of a person would not be possible that way. This is why the blockage of energy channels results in illness or sickness.

In addition, chakras are linked with certain body parts and organs. They impact those organs and give energy to that body part. Hence, chakras enable the human body to function properly by helping organs in performing their tasks with efficiency. Moreover, it is important to remember that every organ is linked to our brain and that our mental health is dependent on our physical health. Mental health is, in turn, linked with our spiritual health. Hence, all of this is interlinked and connected. Each organ in our body has a corresponding point or organ form in the spiritual form. The health of mortal organs has an impact on the immortal counterparts. Chakras or energy centers are not easy to understand as every person has his own chakras meaning that the shape and the performance of chakras vary from person to person. A single shoe cannot fit all feet. Slight modification is required to understand the chakras of every person. Hence, care must be taken when certain exercises are performed to activate the chakras and experts must be cautious about it. Chakras control the behavior of a person as well. For example, if the energy channel of a person that related to self-confidence is blocked in a person, that person will always feel low and bad about his work. He will feel an emptiness and his mood will be overcome his thoughts. He will, hence, act very aggressively towards people who are happy with themselves and their work.

Chakras are known to vibrate at an intensity which is needed in a person's body. Their activity and vibration differs from person to person. In the lower position chakras, vibration is less as compared to the higher position ones. The frequency of vibration at the lower level is less as the lower level chakras are concerned with the emotions of a person. The density of lower level chakras is greater than the higher level chakras. On the other hand, higher level chakras hive more frequency as they are for the brain and mental power.

The well-being of chakras is important for the physical well-being of a person. Chakras bring balance in our lives and their absence leads to sickness, which can end up in death as survival without energy is impossible. It can be seen that people rely on yoga for their physical well-being as well as their spirituality. The reasons for this are that yoga leads to improvement in the health of our chakras. In fact, yoga is performed to polish the chakras of a person. What people do in yoga is to try to bring balance in their chakras and move the lower level chakras to the higher ones. This means that they try to activate their higher level chakras through yoga and meditation. This helps them to bring spirituality in harmony to the mental and physical form. Yoga helps people to find their inner peace and go to a place inside their bodies which is known as the internal space of a person. After the internal space has been created, a person becomes more conscious about how he is spending his energy. This realization helps in keeping a check on personal behavior which ultimately leads to improving the way a person interacts with others in the society. This leads to enabling a person to balance his energy on his own.

An important concept, here, is bringing harmony between the upper and lower level energies. This can be understood with the help of Maslow's pyramid of needs. Maslow presented a model in which he showed a pyramid of needs. The lower level of pyramid was of basic needs of food after which there was another level and this continued upward till the highest level of self-actualization. The theory he presented was that once the lower level needs are fulfilled, the person tries to move up the pyramid to fulfill higher level needs. In the same way, chakras enable a person to move from lower levels of energy to higher ones. Finally, the crown stage is reached which is the highest form of spirituality.

As the higher level energies are less dense than the lower level ones, there is a need to balance this density between the two. An important aspect here is that every level of energy has its counterpart in any other level. For example, the seventh level has its counterpart in first level and sixth with second. This helps in refining the energies to a level where a balance is reached between the two.

Chapter 6: Importance of Centers of Energy

The Sanskrit word chakra denoted a circle or a wheel as has been mentioned before. However, what is important to remember is that these circles represent energy centers in the body. The subtle form of body provides the base for chakras and the subtle body is in itself existing in a non-materialistic form. It can be said that the subtle body is composed of energy itself, whereas the physical form is composed of flesh and bones. The spinning nature and the rotational factor of the energy system give it the name of chakra or wheel. The seven types of chakras mentioned above have their own properties, identity and role. If chakras are seen as a prism, they appear to split the light entering into our body into different colors at different levels of our body. This is the reason behind the association of chakras with specific colors. The need to study chakras arises so that people can master their chakras to unify their personal attributes and to realize the hidden traits in their bodies which are embedded in their soul. By the time a person realizes his chakras, he finds out his own attributes and he reaches a level of spirituality that creates self-awareness.

Conclusion

Thank you again for downloading this book!

I hope this book was able to help you to in understanding Chakras and their significance for life.

The next step is to practice them so that you can actually benefit from this book.

Finally, if you enjoyed this book, please take the time to share your thoughts and post a review on Amazon. It'd be greatly appreciated!

Thank you and good luck!

Book # 2

Zen

The Ultimate Guide to Mastering Zen for Beginners in 60 Minutes or Less!

Table of Contents

Introduction

I want to thank you for downloading the book, "Beginning Zen Buddhism".

In this book you can expect to learn the proven steps and strategies for "Beginning Zen Buddhism"

If you take the time to read this book fully and apply the information held within this book, it will help you to mastering the art of "Zen"

Thanks again for downloading this book, I hope you enjoy it!

Chapter 1: Welcome to Zen Buddhism

Hello and welcome to the world of Zen Buddhism. In this book you will learn how to delve into the world of Buddhism, a slight history of Zen and the topics needed to fully understand the meditation techniques that you will learn.

This book will help you through the beginner phase of Zen Buddhism, where you will transcend the first three Dharma realms and afterwards you will be ready to begin an intermediate course. Buddhism is rich and enlightening way of life that millions of people around the world follow. It is more than just fighting or mystical teachings; it is a guide for many to follow in order to figure out the big questions and the meaning of life. Although, many who start down this path do not reach enlightenment in one life time, they do undergo great spiritual growth and become a better person because of it. Of course if you are not into Zen as a religion, it also has other applications.

Many people in the west use it through forms of Yoga and a means to relax, focus and prepare for the day ahead. Zen is a way for them to separate themselves from the world and transcend it, if only for a moment. If you are looking into this book as a means to get introduced to the religion and you are hoping to take the meditation presented in this book seriously, I ask that you merely use this as a tool instead of a primary mode of knowledge. There are others that are highly trained in the ways of Zen Buddhism such as monks and nuns at monasteries and Zen centers around the world that can help you. As Zen is mainly practiced as a religion in the eastern countries such as China, Japan, Taiwan and Korea; those in the west can find solace in this book, that it does introduce many of the things you will have to learn and teaching you will have to read. Using this book in conjunction with outside advice will strengthen and enrich your growth.

In about sixty minutes you will be familiar with all the techniques, and topics that those beginning in Zen will be familiar with it. So sit back and enjoy the teachings that have spanned thousands of years. Most of the material in this book has been gathered from Buddhist monks and teachings of the Buddha as well as people well versed in it.

Chapter 2: What is Zen Buddhism?

What is Zen Buddhism?

Well, many people are aware of some of the techniques and rituals involved in Zen because of Yoga, but Zen is more than just sitting and breathing. It is connecting to the world around you, expanding your mind and enlightening your soul. As its name dictates, Zen finds its roots in Buddhism.

Buddhism is a religion derived from Hinduism. It was created by a man born, Siddhartha Gautama. Although Gautama was under house arrest, he often took trips out of the palace. While on these trips he encountered an old man, a sick man and a corpse. Wondering how life could come to such a horrific end, he left the palace, renounced the throne and began searching for the meaning to it all. Through days and weeks of strict meditation and fasting, he reached Nirvana; as he discovered the meaning of life. Gautama had become the Buddha. These keys to understanding life became known as the Four Noble Truths: All Life is suffering; the source of suffering is desire; and to stop suffering you must rid yourself of desire. Now, the Buddha knew that this wasn't an easy thing to accomplish so he created a system to help those on the path; this became known as the Eight Fold Paths consisting of: Right View, Right Intention; Right Speech; Right Action; Right Livelihood; Right Effort, Right Mindfulness; and Right Concentration.

Within Buddhism are two main schools of thought: Mahayana and Theravada. Although no one statement can fully explain one school, the purpose of each is clear. The Mahayana school of Buddhism was founded in China about fifteen centuries ago and focuses on the enlightenment of beings rather than the individual self.

The ideal of is to become a Bodhisattva, or someone that has generated Bodhicitta or the idea that spontaneous wish to attain enlightenment and is determined to do so for the benefit of all sentient beings. Bodhisattva strives to eliminate all things from the cycle of life and death. One of the main ideas behind Bodhicitta is the anatman, the sense of self. This is where the schools of Mahayana and Theravada differ.

The teachings of Mahayana believe that the individual self is an illusion.

There is no self, as the elements of the world and the people in it are one. In order for the ideal to be truly reached all sentient beings must be enlightened together, since we cannot separate ourselves from each other. This void of the intrinsic self is known as shunyata or emptiness.

Zen Buddhism is a school of Mahayana, thus shares the same principle of the void of intrinsic self. The word Zen is actually Japanese; its original Chinese name is Ch'an. Zen has different names all over Asia as in Vietnam it's called Thien, and in Korea it's called Seon; so the sense of the enlightenment of all is felt across the world. The exact origin of Zen is traced back to an Indian Sage

Bodhidharma, the first patriarch of Zen. He taught at the Shaolin Monastery of China. The origin of Zen is tied tightly with philosophical Taoism.

The Zen that we know today was crafted by the Sixth Patriarch, Huineng. He shed most of the vestigial Indian properties, allowing the religion to become more Chinese. Because of this, some consider Huineng to be the true father of Zen, not Bodhidharma.

Bodhidharma described Zen as:

A special transmission outside the scriptures;

No dependence on words and letters;

Direct pointing to the mind of man;

Seeing into one's nature and attaining Buddhahood.

Zen is not an intellectual discipline that can be learned from books; rather, practice is necessary to master its principles. It is a practice of studying the mind and seeing into one's nature. This is all done with what possibly is the most important tool in Zen Buddhism, the zazen.

Zazen is a method of meditation used by Zen and the main tool to reaching enlightenment. It is the heart of Zen is requires daily practice. Basic zazen can be learned from the internet, books and videos. However, to attain good form it is rec commended that you meditate in a group every once in a while, as most people finds that it enriches the experience. Zen centers and monasteries aren't as common in the west as it is the east, so you would probably want to just find a group of laypeople and sit together in a common room.

Beginners of zazen are taught to meditate via their breathing, although it isn't the only way. This usually helps with concentration. After you get past this stage you are ready to try sitting for longer periods of time, performing shikantaza (just sitting) or to preform koans with a master. This is a good time to ask for guidance and approval in what you are doing, as well as any other questions. These private interviews are called dokusan.

All around the world, especially in the west, Zen is known as an ancient art of meditation that is mostly used for fighting (kung-fu) and deep spiritual growth. Although Zen Buddhism is used for both, it is important to note that main goal of Zen is to realize the void of self and to help others reach the point of enlightenment so all can be enlightened. This is a long and strenuous journey, not on the body of course, but on the mind. Zazen must be cultivated and appreciated before any real steps can be taken. It is not merely a form of meditation to do in order to become enlightened or to get further down the path; doing that undermines the point. Zazen doesn't have an end goal, not to become enlightened or to reach some deep spiritual connection. Please don't misunderstand, it is used to attain both of these things, but at its core, it is used to train the mind. Through this understanding and experience with the mind, you will be able to perform the exercises that you will learn in this book.

Chapter 3: Getting Started

Now that we know about the history of Zen Buddhism, nailing down exactly what it is and what can be accomplished with it; we are going to get started on the actual practices of Zen Buddhism.

An important thing to note about Zen is that there are two things that one must do in order to succeed in it; study attentively the texts of the Buddha and the monks as well as daily meditation. The teachings will help you on your path and the meditation, zazen, will aid your growth. In this section we will go over how to practice zazen, where to practice it, and the topics that go along with it all, mainly the ten dharma realms, and the seven factors of enlightenment. These teachings will coincide with the types of meditation learned in the next few chapters.

Before we begin zazen we first need to set up a station for it. As stated earlier you can practice zazen in a public place such as a monastery, Zen Center or with a group of people. However, because many beginners have trouble getting into the rhythm of zazen it is recommended that you practice on your own first before joining others. This will allow you to get comfortable and allow you to concentrate for longer periods of time. When you can stay in zazen for about thirty minutes, then you can move on to practicing in a public place.

Creating a zendo or meditation hall, is pertinent in beginning zazen. Zendos are described as small areas dedicated to meditation. They usually have a shelf, high on the wall that holds a Buddha statue. Please be mindful that the statue isn't merely decoration and that it is the highest thing in the room. Adjacent to it, on the left and right sides, are flowers. The flowers, starting off healthy and robust, then wilting, withering and dying, represents impermanence. Fake flowers can be used in place of live ones if you are worried about purposely killing flowers needlessly; as long as the idea of impermanence is still in your mind when gazing upon them. Other zendos include a Buddha statue on a lower table that holds candles and a bowl of sand or rice (to hold the incense). Before the arrangement is a large square cushion, known as the zabuton, and one smaller round one known as the zafu; these are arranged directly in front of the table. Note, that there is no one way to create a zendo, the above descriptions merely describe formal zendos that are usually found in homes and that are similar to the ones in monasteries and zen centers. If few of the above mentioned objects are unavailable, try to at least have the cushion, placed about a foot or so from the wall. This place is to be a special dedicated place where you will come to practice right away.

When sitting on the cushions you can either take the lotus or the half lotus positions, these are the classic zazen position. The lotus position has you sitting, cross-legged on the cushion with the feet placed above your thighs. If you are having trouble visualizing it, the position is similar to sitting "Indian-style". Once this is done, place your hands by your navel, resting on your waist; your fingers from your left hand should be touching the fingers on your right hand and the point of your thumbs should also be touching. In the end, you make an oval with your hands and place them by your navel, resting on your waist.

This is the classic full lotus position. If you cannot get your legs into the full lotus, that's ok, try then for the half lotus, in which you only fold your left or right leg; alternating as you meditate. Most people have trouble getting into the full lotus position, so if you are having trouble that is fine.

Another position known as the seiza position. This position is a bit easier to do than the lotus, as you sit with your legs folded and your feet beneath you. There are benches to help you stay into this position; of course, you can also do it without one. During all of these positions the hands stay exactly the same. Please note that if you are going to use a seiza bench to help you into the position you need to use one according to your height, as that is the way they are made.

If either of the aforementioned positions is difficult for you to get into or stay in for a long period of time, you could always use a chair. When using a chair, your back must not be touching the back rest and your feet must be on the floor. As mentioned above, your hands stay in the same position. The back and neck must be straight for all positions. Because this all seems very meticulous, it is important to practice at home before going to a public meeting. For a more comprehensive guide on getting into positions refer to The Three Pillars of Zen.

Lastly, the main areas that we will be focusing on when going through the steps of beginning Zen Buddhism will be addressing the first three realms of Dharma. You should understand what Dharma is before beginning the first step, as it is good to know what you are attempting to do instead of just blindly following the words of a book.

Dharma is the universal truth common to all individuals at all times that was proclaimed by the Buddaha. Spiritually, Dharmas is used to explain the elements that compose the empirical world. The Dharma Realms are:

1 - Hell

2 - Ghost

3 - Animal

4 - Asura

5 - Man

6 - Deva

7 - Sravaka

8 - Praetyka-Buddha

9 - Bodhisattva

10 -Buddha

In the next chapter we will begin discussing the first steps of training that are told through the story of the ox. As you will learn in your studies, much of Zen is taught through metaphor and allegories. In this book we will rise out of the first few Dharma realms. In order to do this we will be guided by the seven factors of enlightenment:

1. Mindfulness (sati).
2. Investigation of states (dhammavicaya).
3. Energy, vigor (viriya).

4. Joy (piti).

5. Tranquility (passaddhi).

6. Concentration (samadhi).

7. Equanimity (upekkha).

Chapter 4: Seeking the Ox

Now we begin the first step in Zen. The first step is known as Seeking the Ox. We do this by practicing Present Moment Awareness. Present Moment Awareness is exactly how it sounds. It involves living precisely in the moments that pass us by without thinking about the future or about the past. In order to accomplish this we use Mindfulness, one of the steps in the seven factors of enlightenment. Present Moment Awareness is the basis for all Zen Buddhism, so it is important that this step is carried out successfully before moving on.

Before you begin, you should know that there are two steps to learning Mindfulness; one is present moment awareness while the other is cultivating happiness. It may seem strange, but in order to leave the tenth dharma level (where we must begin), we have to defeat ignorance. Ignorance is the source of all ill will, and unhappiness. One does not simply hate ignorance because that is also a negative feeling, in order to cultivate happiness one has to let go of all unwholesome things and ingest only wholesome things. That is part of the purpose of Buddhism, to release unwholesome things and to ingest wholesome things.

Happiness, like everything, is inside of us. That is why we must cultivate it. Happiness can be attained through a variety of ways, from doing generous things such as donating to a charity or simply smiling. It is up to you how you choose to gather your happiness. However, in order to attain happiness you must not do anything unwholesome or acts of cruelty. These acts of cruelty can only be done if you see the people these acts are done upon as the other. Be mindful that there is no other and to think like that undermines the fundamental belief that we are all together and that there is no individual; to believe in doing cruel acts to another is not mindful and one must be mindful to proceed.

Be mindful that everything is inside of you. Being unable to leave the tenth dharma realm because of unwholesome thought is something that you must release and that no one can really help you with. For it is you that set yourself there and only you can release yourself. The tenth dharma level is filled with world of desires, this must be abolished. The other step is to practice present moment awareness. After reading the steps below, you should go to your zendo and practice for as long as you can, but if you go over thirty minutes you can stop if you wish. The three rules to present moment awareness is stated by meditating on the following instructions:

1. Forget the past;

2. Drop thoughts of the future; and

3. Experience only the present moment.

The preliminaries for beginning meditation are listed below:

1) Sit facing a wall with your eyes slightly open and unfocused. Look down, but keep your head erect. This is the classic Zen meditation posture.

2) Do not move while sitting. If the body is moving the mind is moving.

3) Sit in either the lotus or half lotus position; whichever you can accomplish at this point.

4) Keep your eyes slightly open. They must be closed enough to not focus on anything, but wide enough to see if a hand is held in front of it.

5) If you can stay aware while your eyes are closed, you may do so; but you must continue to be awake.

While you sit there instruct your mind to do the aforementioned instructions: Forget the past, drop thoughts of the future and experience only the present moment. As you sit, feel free to listen to the diegetic sound around you; the birds flying by your window, the car passing on the street, the busy chatter of people on their phones, the wind rushing past your window and by your ear, the subtle thuds of people stepping above you or below you if you are in a building, even the breaths (if you can hear it) of the people around you. These sounds are in the moment and if you are focusing on them you are focusing on the present moment.

In addition to this, you should breathe rhythmically. As you breathe count your breaths. Although you can hear the sounds around you and your mind will be racing with thoughts, you mustn't let your mind wander too much or get distracted. To aide you in concentration, focus on counting your breaths. Count your breaths to ten then start over. There isn't a real goal to this. Doing this will not get you closer to enlightenment (at least not like how getting better at this skill will somehow make you reach enlightenment faster), but it will aid in your concentration. Every time you get distracted, go over ten, forget which number you are on or anything else you do that disrupts the pattern, start over from one and begin counting again. Note that you don't breathe so you can count an exhalation, you are breathing normally you are just counting the breaths that you take. If the breath is long, feel free to extend the number as it happens (for example for a long exhalation count siiiixxxx, seeevvveen, etc). Don't congratulate yourself for getting to number ten, just start over at one.

As stated earlier, this dharma that we start in is filled with ill-will things as it is controlled by your mind. These nefarious roots are, as stated by the Buddha as, greed, hatred, and delusion or ignorance. We tend to avoid things that we hate, and tend to run towards things that we want; these are viewed as hatred and greed respectively. Ignorance stems from being ignorant of The Four Noble Truths (which can be found in the previous chapter if you don't know what it is). Thus, we have completed learning the necessary steps for finding the ox. Once we are done here we begin the next step of finding the Footprints of the Ox.

Chapter 5: Finding the Footprints

Now that we have sought out the Ox, we have to find its footprints. This can be thought of as finding a path to follow. In this section we will discuss the ninth level of dharma that we have found ourselves in since we left the tenth level with Present Moment Awareness. In this dharma, we discover a realm of ill-will that can be directly combated with the meditation that we will learn. This meditation will seem very easy to do as you might have done it already as we all may have done it at one time or another when we are going to work, lying down for bed or when we may simply be going about our daily lives.

Probably the most well practiced and well known Zen Buddhist meditation is the loving kindness or Metta meditation. It is one that people all around the world seem to have caught onto in one way or another. The Loving Kindness meditation involves you thinking about the well-being of others. We think about them being well off and begin the mantras that they are happy calm and peaceful. This is done in the zazen posture and typically follows the feelings of happiness cultivated in the Present Moment Awareness meditation. While in this state one must mentally repeat each of the following statements in a similar manner as *"May I be well, happy, calm, and peaceful"*:

May all of the members of my family be well, happy, calm, and peaceful.

May all of my relatives be well, happy, calm, and peaceful.

May all of my friends be well, happy, calm, and peaceful.

May all strangers be well, happy, calm, and peaceful.

May the people I dislike be well, happy, calm, and peaceful and may my dislike fade away.

May all beings on the earth be well, happy, calm, and peaceful.

May all beings throughout all of the universes be well, happy, calm, and peaceful.

The dislike of others and the hatred of said others allows you to fall in the ninth dharma realm, known as the realm of hungry ghost. Here lie the beings that can never be satisfied, they are anxious and live in an environment filled with illusion and fear. Their dissatisfaction comes from not being able to have what they truly want (for instance, one of the ghost is hungry, and has a huge appetite, but has an incredibly small throat that is incapable of really swallowing anything). Because some parts of the hungry ghost realm is ambiguous, it is best to think of it as a transitional period between the hell worlds and the dharma realm of animals. The hungry ghosts have achieved a level of happiness to escape the tenth level, but lack the love and compassion to enter the seventh. They are defiled. Cultivating feelings of hatred and greed begins to drag you back down to the realm of animals, so it is best to avoid such things.

So, each day we practice the Love and Kindness meditation by sitting quietly and letting all thoughts of love and kindness pervade ourselves and the universe. By doing this we are practicing the third level of the six perfections or, the Perfection of Patience. although unrelated, this is akin to the ancient proverb, Love is Patient; where it does not question and hopes that the love present will eventually lead to balance and guides you to the answer that you seek. As we climb out of the ninth dharma level we begin to see the footprints of the Ox.

Traditionally, the second step of finding the footprints of the Ox is seen sort of as a drafting of sots. Usually those that have preserved and those that have successfully overcome the desire to quit are seen in this path. As we go along, the physical pain of meditation subsides a bit and we are becoming more experienced. Those that have quit at this point are left behind, but we do begin to realize that we are all of the same mind and thus the same person. Now, we leave behind our old selves as we have become committed to following the ox until we have caught it.

Although we have made progress we have yet to reach Jhana, a state of complete and utter concentration and stillness; where we become fully immersed in the world around us and transcend ever so slightly to catch a glimpse of the Ox. This, second meditation is a perfect segue into the third meditation technique we learn in which we do see the Ox for the first time, even if it is fleeting. Please note that, that although this book is covering the steps rather quickly and you may think that you can just begin the Present Awareness Meditation, then swing into the Loving Kindness meditation and finally reach the last meditation covered in this book, but let me tell you that that should not be the case. For each of these steps, as a reminder, you should remember that mastering or at least becoming somewhat proficient in these steps requires days of meditation in their subjective techniques.

Do not spend merely a few minutes on the Present Moment Awareness before moving on to this one and do not spend few moments on this one to move on to the next one.

I emphasis this point as the length of the book might show that mastering the meditation techniques is a very easy thing to do. I'm not going to say that it is the hardest thing in the world, it can be done, and yes you can spend a little time trying all of them at first if you'd like; however, if you want to be proficient in it and take it seriously, you need to dedicate the time; however, this book is merely a taste of Zen Buddhism not a full teaching. With that said, if either of these practices hold, unto itself, some sort of merit, please feel free to solely to that practice; but do heed my efforts as we move onto the third technique which is the first technique that helps you achieve that first Jhana experience.

Chapter 6: First Glimpse of the Ox

Finally we come to the third meditation technique known as Silent Present Moment Awareness. It is here that we catch the first glimpse of the Ox and leave the eighth dharma realm. As we transition from the Loving Kindness meditation, we let the love and kindness towards all sentient things is our last thought and we enter silence. This silence is a silence of the mind, we sit in the same position, but we think of absolutely nothing. This is known as true silence and when it is achieved the Ox may be seen. While in this form, really try to clear your mind of all thoughts; even thoughts that are thinking about what you are doing. So don't think "I'm going to enjoy this morning" or, "I am beginning Silent Present Awareness", just stop thinking all together; let your mind be at ease as you shut it down. If you are having trouble with this it is good to follow the instructions of a Yoshi or teacher; if a teacher is not available, and then try looking for text such as the Spectrum of Consciousness by Ken Wilbur to help you along.

As we move into this, we objectify ourselves and the voice from that commands our true self to speak. The silence is there to allow our true self to come out and speak. After a while you may experience a bit of enlightenment like Roshi Philip Kapleau, the founder of the Rochester Zen Center:

"All at once the roshi, the room, every single thing disappeared in a dazzling stream of illumination and I felt myself bathed in a delicious, unspeakable delight...For a fleeting eternity I was alone—I

alone was...Then the roshi swam into view. Our eyes met and flowed into each other, and we burst out laughing..."

It is at this point that people begin to believe that their training is over. They have experienced quite a vision and now they think they are ready to move on. These people usually believe that they saw God or transcended even higher than the Buddha, but that is simply not the case. After this experience we are ready to go deeper into Buddhism and can begin practicing it to its fullness every day. As time goes on the moment and bliss of seeing the ox for the first time will pass, and you will begin to calm down. Many painting of the Ox exist to show that the experience is mind-blowing and overwhelming. With this we have grown out of the eighth dharma level and risen above the realm of animals. It is at this point that the repentance gatha can begin to be said and a vow to renounce all evil actions.

Some people that leaves the world and becomes a monk or a nun. This should be done before any heavy responsibility is taken in the world such as getting married or having children. It is not too uncommon to see men and women leave behind their spouses and kids to lead lives in the monastery. If you are going to take Zen Buddhism that seriously, I suggest leaving this book behind to search for a better source of knowledge, unless you are just using this as a means of introduction, which, if you are, then please proceed.

Every day you are to repeat the Repentance Gatha as it reinforces the works that we do and is a nice way to wrap up the first three meditations. The repentance gatha is more or less the following:

"We can renounce ill will, greed, animal cruelty/meat-eating, drinking, desires for wealth and fame, etc., and any other activity that conflicts with the precepts."

Small ways to ensure this is to not stuff yourself when you eat, and to practice generosity by giving to worthy charities. One way to begin living your life closer to the Theravada monk (yes, it is a different school of Buddhism than Zen, but that doesn't matter in this case), is to eat one vegetable meal per day, before noon and to drink tea in the afternoon and evening. With each passing day our happiness increases and loving kindness increases, diminishing ignorance in its wake. To practice generosity you can donate to a Tzu Chi organization. They are similar to the American Red Cross, but they are founded on Buddhist transition. The money is spent on food that doesn't from animals and they have relief organizations around the world. The donations of the organization are deposited once a year on the Chinese New Year. If you don't live near ta Tzu Chi center, they can send you a donation container that serves as a piggy bank. You can put whatever amount you wish into the container, a few pennies or whatever you feel is necessary. Don't misunderstand that this is something that is required of you. Unlike Christian religions, it is not like the collection plate, where you have to donate a certain amount every week.

If you don't want to send money to the organization then try being generous in other ways, give money to a homeless person, volunteer at a soup kitchen, babysit the child of a single mother or father so they can have a break for the night. Anything that you deem as a generous act, it can be done towards another person.

And that concludes our small tutorial on the ways of Zen Buddhism. I hope you enjoyed yourself and that this was a useful tool to help bring you into the world. If you are serious about doing this, I suggest going through the book more slowly, learning more from outside materials, but use this book as a tool to help with the meditation. The meditations and steps shown here is only the beginning after becoming proficient enough, you should move on to more intermediate steps where you will rise higher through the dharma realms, and hopefully one day reach nirvana. Until then, I hope you enjoyed our little foray into the world of Zen Buddhism and I hope it serves you well in the future.

Conclusion

Thank you again for downloading this book!

I hope this book was able to help you to *Beginning Zen Buddhism.*

Once you've completed this book in full the next step is to seek an intermediate course.

Finally, if you enjoyed this book, please take the time to share your thoughts and post a review on Amazon. It'd be greatly appreciated!

In addition please be sure to take a look on the next page as I have provided you with more high quality books I've published which I'm certain can help you out a ton!

Thank you and good luck on your journey!

Book # 3

Reiki

The Ultimate Guide to Mastering Reiki for Beginners in 30 minutes or Less!

Table of Contents

Introduction

I want to thank you and congratulate you for downloading the book, "Reiki-The Ultimate Guide to Mastering Reiki for Beginners in 30 minutes or less!"

This book contains proven steps and strategies for learning Reiki and understanding it completely

If you take the time to read this book fully and apply the information held within this book will help you to start using Reiki to self-heal and then use it to heal others.

Thanks again for downloading this book, I hope you enjoy it!

Chapter 1: An Introduction to Reiki

Reiki is the accent art of healing by using the laying on of hands. The person who is administering the healing becomes a vessel for the healing energy addressing physical, mental, emotional and spiritual issues that the recipient is dealing with.

Before we go any further, I want to explain that this can be very dangerous for the person practicing Reiki. When you practice Reiki you have to open yourself up to the healing energies. This can also open you up to much other energy as well. Those who are not experienced can allow negative energies to come into them and although this will not harm the recipient it has been known to cause many issues in the person who is practicing's life.

Many people will tell you that you do not have to worry about protecting yourself when you are practicing but that you need to make sure you are balance. While I do believe that it is very important to be balanced within oneself when practicing Reiki, I also believe it is important to set up a barrier so that if any negative energy were trying to come your way you would be safe from any harm.

It is just like when a psychic prepares for a session, they know they are going to encounter good but on the off chance any negative comes their way the prepare for it beforehand. You can choose not to protect yourself and that is completely up to you but this next little bit is for those who would like some protection.

The first thing you need to do is choose a spiritual path and follow it. I am not going to get into a discussion on the different paths and opinions on each but you have to understand that Reiki is a very spiritual process therefore you need to ground yourself in a spiritual belief. This does not mean that you have to become a saint over night, what it means is that you try.

Once you have chosen a spiritual path you are going to pray for protection from every negative energy that would try to come against you. While you are healing, if you feel anything negative coming toward you, you should focus on a sacred object from whatever spiritual path you have chosen.

Finally after the session is over you need to break all ties with any negative energy that may have come upon you.

Many people who practice Reiki inadvertently take on the issues of the person they are healing so if you are healing someone with a mental disorder you need to physically speak out that you break any ties with mental disorders and you do not allow them in your life.

It may seem a little strange at first but you will get used to speaking these things out. And since you are practicing Reiki to begin with you probably already understand they type of havoc negative energy can wreak on a persons life.

You also need to understand that you do not control the healing Reiki energy. Therefore you are going to be unable to tell someone you are going to help them with a specific issue. You see, a person may come to you with a physical issue or you may try to heal yourself of a specific physical issue only to find that it has not been affected. The Reiki energy goes to where it is need most in the body, bringing complete balance.

So if you are going to practice Reiki you need to explain to people that you cannot heal a specific problem but the Reiki energy will heal what is needed the most. It works like this, if someone came into my home and stated that they needed physical healing because they were always tired, the Reiki energy then finds that they are depressed therefore needing mental or emotional healing in order to bring balance to their lives. The Reiki energy would work on the depression and not the symptom of feeling tired.

Often times this discourages people but if it is explained beforehand they tend to be more accepting of the healing no matter what it is.

Chapter 2: Clearing Your Energy Field

Before you can perform a Reiki session, you have to clear your own energy field. If you do not clear your own energy field, most of the energy that is channeled will go toward healing and cleansing your own energy field and not that of your client.

The most important thing you will ever learn from a Reiki class is that you are to work on yourself first. The fact is that those who care for others tend to avoid taking care of themselves. The first rule of Reiki is that if you do not take care of yourself first, you cannot take care of others.

You also need to understand that it is up to you to heal you as it is up to the client to heal themselves. You see if a client comes in asking you to heal them you need to explain to them that you are just a vessel for the energy, they will be harnessing that energy and actually doing the healing themselves.

You need to make sure that you do not just jump into giving others Reiki, this needs to be performed on yourself on a regular basis. The more you do it, the better you will get and the more in tune with the energy you will become. I suggest you actually give yourself Reiki for at least 3-4 months before ever practicing on someone else.

You also need to understand that you're body needs to be as healthy as possible to be the best Reiki provider. If you are not eating healthy foods, drinking a ton of sugary drinks, not exercising and just not taking care of your body you will not be very successful at Reiki.

You need to also focus on your mental, emotional and spiritual state as well as the environment you live in. If you live in a stressful environment and try to work Reiki on others, you will find that it does not work because the energy will again try to heal you first.

So make sure you are taking the time out to meditate, create a calm place at home as well as in the office if you begin using Reiki on others.

Now as I said you need to practice Reiki regularly to clear your own energy field. You need to do this daily and not just when you remember to.

To do self Reiki, you need to start with a relaxing environment. Most people prefer to practice self Reiki first thing in the morning when they wake up and in the evening when they are going to bed.

Make sure you have a calm, relaxing environment, you can also have a soothing recording that you listen to while you practice Reiki. Next you need to make sure you are in a comfortable position and have a set plan. You need to work down your plan in the same pattern every day. It will look something like this:

- *Top of Head*

- *Face*

- *Neck*

- *Chest*

- *Abdomen*

And work your way down as far as you want to go all the way to your feet if you would like. Then you will work backwards from your feet all the way back up to the top of your head or whatever starting point you have chosen.

You will take your hands and place them either on or right over the area you are working on. Hold them for a set length of time, two minutes seems to work great. You can use a small timer to track the time spent on each part of your body.

While you have your hands placed on or right above each area, focus on your breathing as well as whatever sensations you are feeling at the moment. If you finish one area but feel drawn to go back, repeat that area until you are comfortable removing your hands and moving on to the next area.

You want to do this for at least 3 to 4 months daily before ever practicing Reiki on someone else. Again you need to make sure you do this daily, I understand that there are times when you may not be able to fit in an entire session but some Reiki is better than no Reiki at all. If you can only focus on a few parts than make sure you focus on the ones you feel most drawn to. Either way, the Reiki energy is going to find the part of your body that it needs to work on at that moment.

While you are practicing Reiki on yourself, you will find that thoughts will come and go, allow them to but stay focused on your breathing, if a negative thought enters your mind, push it out and refocus. You may find that thoughts of what you have to accomplish that day or what bills need paid or even the random thought of what you need to purchase at the grocery store will try to creep into your mind, if it does let it pass, you can focus on those thoughts later but for now you need to be focused completely on balancing yourself.

As these thoughts enter your mind, just remind yourself that you are becoming balanced, you are healed and go back to focusing on your breath.

I have spoken to many people who have stated that in just one week of using self Reiki they have seen amazing changes in their lives. Some say that they just feel more positive and that they are able to think more clearly, others state they have become more productive and are much happier with life in general while still others say that in only a week they are seeing symptoms of health problems they have suffered with for years just disappear.

Before we go any farther, I want to make it clear that at no point should you quit taking any prescribed medications, it is okay to add some vitamins and minerals if a doctor says it is okay but until the doctor takes you off of your medications, continue taking them.

Chapter 3: How to Start Helping Others

Before we go any further, I want everyone to understand that Reiki is not a religion, it was never a religion and it is used by people of many different religions. Just like meditation or positive affirmations it is a way to bring balance into your life with the added benefit of healing your energy fields so that your body is healed as well.

Reiki does not infringe upon any religion and you may need to explain this to those who are asking for your help because if they feel as if they are doing something wrong the Reiki energy will focus on correcting the way they feel and not balancing out what is really wrong.

There are also those who believe if they use Reiki they are opening themselves up to psychic abilities or communication with the other side. This is because back in the 80's there was a book written by a woman who claimed that her students began seeing their spirit guide after using Reiki. Reiki is not going to give you any psychic abilities nor is it going to open you up to communicating with the other side, it is simply an exchange of healing energy.

Reiki is not a form of massage therapy. There are massage therapists that will offer Reiki sessions to their clients but Reiki does not involve any manipulation of bones or tissue. In fact you don't have to touch your clients when you are using Reiki, you can simply hover your hands above the person.

I also want you to understand that Reiki does not deplete the energy of the practitioner. Many people have believed this for a long time but the fact is that when you are a practitioner of Reiki, you are just channeling the energy, it is not your personal energy that is being used. If a person who is using Reiki feels tired after they have worked with a client it is usually because something is out of balance within themselves which is one more reason to make sure you are doing your daily self Reiki.

Once you have tuned in to Reiki, you may begin having a sense of peace and calmness, you may feel strangely positive, and may even start to have very vivid dreams. It is okay if you do not feel anything different right away this will come with time. When you begin feeling a change in your life you know you are ready to help others.

Before I begin explaining how really simple it is to help others by using Reiki, I want to talk a little bit about opening a practice. Many people once they begin being able to help those around them decide to open a Reiki practice in their home or outside of their home. While the purpose of using Reiki is not about making money it is understandable that you would want to charge a fee for your time.

What I want to make sure you understand is that you need to make sure you are actually helping people before you start charging an hourly rate for your services. Practice on yourself of course but also practice on your children or your friends. No harm will come to anyone who uses Reiki so you do not have to worry about getting it wrong. What you do need to worry about is giving people a false sense of hope when they come to you. If you do not have enough experience you will literally be taking their money and not providing them with any service.

Now on to helping those around you. Like I said I want you to practice self Reiki for at least 3 to 4 months and then you can begin practicing on your friends and family.

Reiki is actually very simple and I know it may seem complicated when you first begin but it really is not. Once you practice for a little while when you lay your hands on someone or something with the intent to heal them the energy will naturally flow through you. This really should take no effort on the part of the practitioner.

You do not have to perform any elaborate ritual when you begin a Reiki session, although some to bring their hands to their heart and bow in reverence to Reiki and asking Reiki to flow through them. You do not have to ask for Reiki to flow through you but it is out of respect that some do this.

When you begin using Reiki on someone you should not promise them specific results. As I said earlier Reiki goes where it is needed most and often this is very unpredictable. Instead tell your clients that Reiki will help them in the way that will benefit them the most because after all that is the truth.

When you place your hands on or above the person you are working with, it is not uncommon for the both of you to feel hot or cold sensations, vibrations, or tingling. Often times when the practitioner is feeling the sensation of heat, the receiver will feel a cold sensation so do not worry if your client is experiencing the opposite of what you are.

There are also times when the receiver will not feel a sensation in the moment but will feel it later in the day or even a few days later. And there will also be times when the receiver will feel no sensations at all but neither of you should worry because as long as you have put in the time to practice you can rest assured that Reiki is benefiting the client.

Chapter 4: Forgiveness

There may be times when your or the client neither one feel as if anything has taken place. This is because the power of Reiki is very dependent on the receiver letting go of past hurts and negative thoughts and feeling. These thoughts and feelings may even be subconscious but they have to be released.

If this happens you need to provide a bit of counseling to your client, direct them toward positive thinking and positive living, refer them to a good councilor if you feel you cannot help them move past the issues and explain to them that these issues are holding them back from receiving the benefits of Reiki.

Often times you can feel it when you lay your hands on a person, sometimes when you enter the room with the person you can feel it if the negativity is strong enough.

One thing I have seen done is that a questionnaire is filled out before each session asking questions like:

- *Do you harbor any un-forgiveness against anyone for any reason?*

- *Do you feel that you are a mostly positive or mostly negative person?*

There were a total of about 10 questions reworded but trying to get the same answer of whether the client was holding onto any negative feelings. If they are you may want to talk to them before the session and explain how the negativity affects the power of Reiki.

You can offer them a free MP3 or even CD discussing positive affirmations and living a positive life and explain that this is just part of the process.

You can also explain to them that they can go ahead and go through a Reiki session and the energy may help work out these deep issues or negative thoughts they are holding onto. While Reiki works on the deeper issues, they may see a reduction in the symptoms they are having to deal with but this can cause the process to take longer than it would if they worked on forgiveness and positive living.

If you find that what you were once doing does not seem to be working for your clients and that your self Reiki is not as strong as it used to be you may feel that your Reiki energy is diminishing. The fact is that the energy you receive is there for life what has happened is that you have an area of your life that has become unbalanced.

Many people give up Reiki when this happens because they really do not understand what is going on. I want to make sure that if this happens to you that you understand what is happening and do not stop helping others with Reiki, all you have to do is figure out a way to rebalance your life. Sometimes this may mean taking some time away from practicing Reiki on others and focusing only on self Reiki once again or it may mean dealing with a negative situation in your life that you have allowed to go on for too long.

Either way if you feel your Reiki diminishing, understand this is not a punishment or the end for you. It is just unbalance in your life.

I spoke briefly earlier about a practitioner taking on the clients symptoms. This is another reason why people become discouraged and stop practicing. The only time you will take on another persons symptoms is when you allow yourself to. You see nothing happens in our lives unless we allow it to happen. If you have strong feelings for the client or a desire to help them with a specific issue you may find that you are taking on their symptoms just to make them happy. This often happens with those who work with very sick loved ones.

This also happens to those who feel like they have to prove that they really can help their clients. Instead of letting Reiki work through them, they are often trying to force something to happen, when they try to control the Reiki energy it opens them up to taking on the negativity of the client. The only way to deal with this is to never feel like you have to produce results, this is the job of Reiki, remember you are just a vessel for the energy, it is not you who is doing the healing.

There are also symbols that can be used from accent Reiki that are said to prove protection for those who are unable to stop themselves from taking on their clients symptoms. What you would do is draw a power symbol in the palm of each hand before each session.

I tend to steer away from this because people are still very leery when it comes to any type of symbol that may contain power and may be scared away from Reiki thinking it is evil.

You can draw the symbol instead on the core of your body which is said to help protect you as well. You can also use affirmations to help with this. Before each session you will have some form of meditation or a ritual that you do for yourself to help you prepare, all you have to do is add to this. You will repeat out loud that you will not take on the negativity of your client, you choose not to allow that negativity to affect you.

It really is that simple. Reiki is not mysterious and it is not magic if you work to keep yourself positive and balanced you can help those who need it.

Chapter 5: Tips

I want to go over a few tips with you than will help you in yourself Reiki sessions as well as sessions with clients.

The first tip I want to give you is that you should never rush a session. Most of the time you want to schedule a 60 minute session but allow yourself up to 90 minutes. Often you will find that Reiki practitioners try to rush through sessions in order to see more clients or they only focus on one specific symptom trying to treat it. This is not how Reiki works, make sure you take the time needed with each client. Some may not need a long period of time other will need longer sessions. Don't be greedy with Reiki.

Make sure when you are working with clients that you practice good hygiene. You are going to be in close contact with many different people and you want to make sure that your personal hygiene is up to par. You also want to make sure that you are washing your hands and your table after seeing each client. You don't want people spreading germs and clients getting sick every time they visit you.

Before you start a session with a client if you are going to be physically placing your hands on them you need to ask permission to do so. You also need to do whatever you can to keep your clients comfortable. You will be going over their entire body and this includes what some would call private areas on their body. Before you place your hands on these areas you need to ask your clients permission. An alternative is to hover your hands above the area but make sure the client knows what you are doing.

Often a client will become uncomfortable having someone's hands close to these areas. Another thing you can do is have the client place their hands over the area and hover your hand above theirs if it makes them feel more comfortable. Reiki is able to travel through their hands and able to travel the short distance from your hands hovering over their hands as well so they will not lose any benefit.

Do not skip these areas of the body just because it may make you are the client feel uncomfortable. The entire body needs to be focused on during a session and if you skip over any are the client will not receive all of the benefits they could from Reiki. If the client requests that you skip these areas make sure they understand they are missing out on some of the benefits of Reiki.

To get a lot of experience, offer to volunteer your services at a local hospital or nursing home. You will be bettering your skills while helping others as well.

Don't focus on charging a fee for Reiki sessions when you first start out. It is much more important that you focus on getting the experience that you need.

Continue with Reiki education. There are three levels of Reiki practitioners, one, two and three. The final level is a Reiki Master. There are courses you can take to move up in the levels and learn more and more about Reiki. As you move up in the levels you will be able to help more people. It is best to go to a Reiki Master for complete training. You can of course go to someone on one of the other levels but they will not be able to get you to a master level. Deciding how far you want to go though is completely up to you.

You can also create a personal Reiki box. To do this you will take a crystal and put it in a box with a lid, you will draw Reiki symbols on the inside of the box and place your intentions inside. You can place anything from becoming more productive to healing of heart disease to getting a specific amount of money. It is basically using Reiki, just as you would positive affirmations. You will do Reiki over the box for five minutes and from that moment on the box is activated. You can check your intentions once a week and tear up the ones that have been accomplished. You can also burn them releasing them to the universe.

A Reiki notebook can also be created. Again you will draw the Reiki symbols, and do a five minute Reiki over the notebook once this is complete the notebook is activated and you can write your requests in it.

Share the Reiki box or notebook with clients, family and friends. It will make your job much easier when they are in a session with you.

I stated earlier that you could work with a Reiki Master in order to fully learn Reiki but this is not necessary. Reiki is so simple and so safe that even a child can learn it. The great thing is that today many masters are posting videos online for those who want to learn. Once you learn, make sure to share your knowledge with others. As long as we continue to share Reiki, Reiki will continue.

When you begin Reiki, focus on self-healing, use your Reiki box or notebook for only yourself, focus on learning as much as you can about self-healing and once you have mastered that move on to helping others. Take the time you need to master each level and don't try to rush yourself because you want to do more this will only cause you to become frustrated and your Reiki will diminish.

Chapter 6: A Few Final Words

I want to end this book by saying a few final words about Reiki. I know when you are first starting out this can seem almost impossible but if you just give it a chance and preform the self-healing, you will be amazed at what you will experience.

You can clear the energy of a room or home by using Reiki as well. There are those who feel that their home is full of disturbances, these are often caused by a poltergeist which is caused from negative energy that is being suppressed by a person. Many people do not know what to do when these occur and they jump to the idea that their house is haunted. You can offer your services to friend and family that are having negative experiences in their homes. It is also a good idea to use Reiki to clean the energy when you are moving into a new home.

When you are in the middle of a Reiki session with a client, you may notice that as your hands pass over certain places on their body your hands become heavy. You need to focus a little more as you go through your session because this usually means that there is low energy flow in the area or even an energy blockage.

Salt will help contain negative energy. When you are preforming a Reiki session, place a bowl of salt at the foot of the receiver, as you sweep down their body with your hands you are pushing the negative energy into the bowl. Do this three to five times and when the session is over wash the salt down the drain getting all of the negative energy out of the area and away from the person and yourself.

Repeating mantras while you are preforming Reiki can help you keep random thoughts out of your mind. There are traditional mantras you can repeat or you can make something up of your own expressing what you want from the session. For instance: I take total healing energy into myself, or As total healing flows through me I allow it to work for its greater purpose.

Whatever the mantra is that you choose, you should repeat it throughout the entire session, helping you to focus all of your thoughts on the Reiki.

There are those who can reach the level of Reiki master in just a few days, it all depends on how open you are to the process and how much you focus on it. You will not become a master in a few days if you only do one 20 minute self-session and you should not feel discouraged if you are not able to heal others in just a few days. Remember it takes time to become great at anything. Those who master Reiki in a few days are called natural healers, they have been channeling Reiki energy their entire life. For the rest of us it can take some time to master.

Finally, you should not worry if you see variations in Reiki training. The way one person teaches will be completely different from the way another person teaches. One person may focus more on balancing the entire body whereas another person may be a medical healer and focus more on the physical body. It is best if you can have a few teachers whether it be online or in person so that you can see different variations of Reiki and choose the one that works for you.

I hope that you can use everything that you have learned in this book to become a master at Reiki. I also hope that this book has helped you to understand what Reiki really is and what it is not.

Conclusion

Thank you again for downloading this book!

I hope this book was able to help you to get started on your path to using Reiki.

The next step is to focus on self-healing follow what you have learned in the book and you will be well on your way to using Reiki to heal others as well.

Finally, if you enjoyed this book, please take the time to share your thoughts and post a review on Amazon. It'd be greatly appreciated!

Thank you and good luck!

Book 4

Kundalini

A Step by Step Guide to Mastering Kundalini for Beginners in 30 minutes or Less!

Table of Contents

Introduction

I want to thank you and congratulate you for downloading the book, Kundalini: A Step by Step Guide to Mastering Kundalini for Beginners in 30 minutes or Less!

This book contains proven steps and strategies for preparing yourself towards the spiritual journey of unleashing your inner Kundalini energy and mastering Kundalini awakening.

Tell me, where did you hear about kundalini? Did you stumble upon it on some flyer? Perhaps hear it from your neighbor? Did you think you need to go to India or approach some spiritual guru in order to master it?

Worry not! You can start this mystic mission by yourself at your very own home. You do not need to spend hundreds of dollars in paying a spiritual master for something that you can easily learn in this book.

If you take the time to read this book fully and apply the information held within this book will help you understand the role of Kundalini in achieving a better and higher state of consciousness, understand that it is not simply done through chanting and groaning your way through a whole hour of session. Kundalini is a delicate and mystical spiritual path that must be undertaken with faith.

This book will also help you awaken the sleeping serpent within you and reach mystic enlightenment as it isequipped with steps that will guide you in triggering your very own Kundalini phenomenon. The instructions provided for the Kundalini awakening will only take less than 30 minutes.

And this book has more to offer as it also discusses the importance of commitment, meditation and purification in your quest of mastering Kundalini.

Thanks again for downloading this book, I hope you enjoy it!

Chapter 1: Understand Kundalini

Kundalini is not a new mainstream Indian concept. It is not your latest recreational activity introduced in order to give bored individuals something novel to do. Nor is it a new method to lose weight like what others perceive the purpose of yoga is. The history of Kundalini is one filled with mysticism and spirituality. Others consider it to be the way to achieve communion with God or even attain the status of a god. It is a big stride towards spiritual evolution.

Kundalini is described as the spiritual energy dwelling within one's body that must be raised and awakened for you to achieve purification of bodily systems and reach a new state of consciousness.It is the Eastern terminology given to the energy which lies dormant and shown symbolically like a coiled snake wrapped three and a half times at the base of the spine(Kumar & Dempsey, 2002). It exists in everyone's body and lies latent until one is ready for its release or one purposely triggers it. Also known as the libidinal and unconscious force, Kundalini energy lies coiled at the base of the spine in a triangular bone called the sancrum like a sleeping serpent waiting to be awakened. It is one of the components of one's spiritual or "subtle" body along with the chakras or your psychic centers; nadis, the energy channels; bindu, which refers to the drops of essence; and prana, one's subtle energy.

Awakening Kundalini leads to enlightenment and involves the energy moving up from the base of the spine to the top of the head. The manifestation of this progress from its initial location is felt as cool breeze across the palms of your hands or the soles of your feet. However, in the case when the movement of the energy was not properly done and there is an imbalance, this breeze will seem warm across the specified areas. Do you feel a tingle or an electric current running along your spine? Then you must be feeling the movement of the Kundalini, as well. The energy passes through different chakra points which correspond to different levels of awakening and spiritual experience. Reaching the top of the head – the crown – leads to a significant and profound mystical experience. This explains why it's not a one time, big time deal. Quitting after raising Kundalini once is not the proper way to do it. On your first endeavor, you might just activate a lower level chakra point and experience a less significant spiritual experience. Moreover, enlightenment is a gradual and staggered affair. Kundalini must be raised many times before it can fully grow. A single Kundalini experience may occur for at least 5 minutes and at most 30 minutes. This duration may lengthen by training and higher development. It also depends on the energy resources of a person. If his energy is depleted, the experience implicated in Kundalini awakening may not be long.

Arousal through spiritual exercises and even spontaneous circumstances brings out a higher level of one's self. Mystical enlightenment and illumination can be achieved. We have the potential to become better than what we are now. Mastering of Kundalini would aid us in developing a different spiritual version of ourselves without the risk of our personalities being lost. If you fear that your friends will no longer recognize you after mastering

Kundalini, don't fret. The traits and characteristics that made you who you are will not be buried under the new state of consciousness that you will embrace.

When you achieve enlightenment through Kundalini arousal, you will perceive the world differently. This might sound cliché but your life will change as the Kundalini energy within you will remove the veil that's covering your eyes from seeing the world. Like water, you will undergo a purification process that will eradicate the resistance and impurities blocking you from experiencing pure love, and trust, among others.

You will experience a different and more comprehensive understanding of the world and reality. You do not need to take in tablets or shoot powders up your nose anymore in order to achieve ecstasy because spiritual enlightenment would help you achieve that feeling.

Activating the Kundalini circuits is a form of transformation. Imagine yourselfas larvae. It's not something ideal, is it? But once you trigger the bodily changes through Kundalini, you can unleash a new circuit that would make you turn into a butterfly. The body begins to reorganize itself after raising Kundalini and it will adapt a new state of being.

Evenafter a person reverts to his normal self, his consciousness and knowledge returning to its original state as well, after a Kundalini awakening, one's spiritual abilities will remain heightened and enhanced.

There are various ways as to how you can awaken your Kundalini. Gurus and spiritual masters can help as well as meditations, breathing exercises, and mantra chanting. It has been reported though that Kundalini can be spontaneously stimulated after a psychological or physical trauma. However, it is emphasized that awakenings through spiritual exercises are better compared to spontaneous ones. When it is by accident (e.g. trauma, childbirth, near-death experiences), the symptoms resemble those experienced in a true Kundalini awakening but are rather unpleasant and damaging.

There are two main approaches in awakening your Kundalini. On one hand, we have the passive approach wherein you surrender yourself to the ministrations and guidance of a spiritual master or guru. A master who has previously experienced the Kundalini phenomenon is responsible for arousing one's own.

On the other hand, we have the active approach. This book will teach you to take initiative in awakening your own energy. This method would incorporate concentration, breathing, and visualization exercises.

The first thing that you have to do before the inner serpent within you can be stirred to rise is preparation. You must first equip your mind and body with the right knowledge and state of being before you endeavor to open your spiritual channels. And knowing aboutKundalini is a very important step. Time and time again, we hear the saying, "Knowledge is power". Obviously, knowing what one is doing goes a long way in accomplishing it. If you want to try motocross racing, you don't just grab a bike from the nearest garage, turn the engine on and zoom your way into oblivion or at the very least, to the hospital. Without preparation, jumping straight into the fire is risky and dangerous. This is why a person who desires to try to awaken his Kundalini must be taught and educated in this subject matter. At times, people want spiritual development to happen with a snap of their fingers, desperate to reach the acclaimed mystical illumination. But they fail to realize that the risk level of acquiring the negative consequences is proportional to the quality of their preparation.

You must have faith in what awakening the Kundalini will achieve. A cynic who tries to open his energy channels just for the fun of it would not likely succeed in doing so. His belief system must be established first.

In arousing Kundalini, you should also know that chakra centers play very vital roles. There are 6 chakra centers associated in the Kundalini process. These centers will amass energy and once it reaches its peak, energy would be released in an upward flow towards the top of the body, triggering the chakra centers above. A Kundalini phenomenon which is fully raised is called the internal snake phenomenon. When this happens, one feels like as if a literal snake pushes its way up between your anus and genitals. It then travels in a spiral up through the body, pushing your organs and internal body parts out of the way along the process.

For one to raise a full Kundalini phenomenon, one must gather a lot of energy at the base chakra center. Through practice, you can become better in accumulating energy in your centers and once the energy mass reaches critical points, it would be released. One of the physical manifestations of this explosion of energy is a tingle or electrical spike along the spine.

Chapter 2: No One-Night Stands

The next step in your preparation is committing yourself to the journey. Doing Kundalini should not arise from a desire to conform to what other people are doing or because you think it's cool.You also shouldn't do it just so you could have something to post as a Facebook status or tweet. Egoistic tendencies must be eradicated when you want to master Kundalini.

Additionally, awakening the sleeping energy within you requires a commitment in your part to be faithful to the spiritual path. Kundalini isn't just about achieving ecstasy. It's about developing a spiritual consciousness that will transform you as a person.

It also takes commitment to go through the exercises that can arouse your Kundalini energy. You can't just say you've had enough after your first attempt. Quitters are losers. Look at it this way. You enter into a relationship. Without commitment, you'd probably end up breaking it off with your partner after the first few weeks because it has become tiresome and full of hassle. Without commitment, you'd just leave your partner in bed after the first orgasm! It's not a relationship then, but a one-night stand. There is no one-night stand in the case of awakening your Kundalini energy. The spiritual path doesn't encourage the participation of those whose hearts are not into the task.

It is a transformational process that you can't afford to just stop according to your whims. You also need to stand by whatever consequences you will gain as Kundalini has been implicated to have long-term, transformational effects that may be strong enough to change the structure of our DNA, causing changes to even the cells (Lim, ND). In other words, this is serious stuff. There is no joke hidden that you can read between the lines.

Full awakening would probably take a longer time that you have anticipated if you do not take this earnestly. Actually, the length of the process depends on every individual. If you have the necessary mindset and have prepared well, mastering it would not make you break a lot of sweat.

So, ask yourself why you are doing this. Do you believe in Kundalini, in the first place? Did you just do this because you happened to hear your colleague at work speak this foreign word?

If you do believe in it, invest your thoughts into the proper execution of this process and be exacting in the observance of the steps. Don't do anything half-heartedly because it's no better than not doing this at all. Any hesitation or doubt to the experience may lead to complications to your psyche. It may even be permanently damaged because of the mental perspective that you don on while you take this course.

Also, do not allow other people to influence what you believe in. Others might find the whole concept of the Kundalini energy to be preposterous and associate it with another Indian mumbo-jumbo. As long as you have faith, nothing and no other opinion matters. Fact is: you are doing this for yourself and not for them.

Chapter 3: Purification of Desires

Do not let earthly desires occupy your every thought. You want more dollars in your bank account? You want to be more beautiful or successful or popular? That's fine but don't let it fill up every nook and cranny of your mind 24 hours a day. In awakening your Kundalini, you should endeavor to free your minds of impurities such as wants and needs in order to prepare yourself to the energy that will soon be coursing through your body.

In your Kundalini sessions, try not to let thoughts of what you want to eat for dinner interrupt your meditation. The goal of arousing the sleeping energy within you is the achievement of enlightenment and mulling over how fried chicken is so delicious will not help you achieve your endgame.

Furthermore, in order to prepare one's body for a spiritual awakening, detoxifying it from impurities is a must. Our energy flows through our bodies which serve as vehicles. Imagine your spirit energy as the driver and your body as the car. Everything that you do to your car will have consequences on the probability of reaching your destination. The food that you eat which enters your body and the secretions from the glands which leaves it will affect your chakras.

One must consume clean fuel sources – that is, a diet rich in nutrients makes up for a healthy life force. Processed foods will introduce toxins into the vehicle and would only lead to its deterioration. Fruits and vegetables will aid in easier digestion and would not fatigue your body so much. Consumption of junk foods is also discouraged since they definitely do not bring in nutrients into your body and can just create organ complications. Take note that what you eat is the fuel of your car. Imagine that instead of gasoline which is the proper source of energy needed to run your car, you feed it with orange juice or muddy water. OJ can't make your vehicle run and not only that.It would most likely destroy some parts of your car.

Likewise, your body needs the proper sources of energy. Not everything that is edible is appropriate.

Additionally, drinking plenty of water is not only beneficial for your physical body but also for your spiritual one. Avoid drinking alcoholic beverages. Most importantly and obviously, do not partake in any alcoholic drink as you are about to engage in a Kundalini session because it will mess with your energy centers and with the clarity of your thoughts.

One should also abstain from drugs. Not only do these substances create negative effects on the physical body, they also lead to the deterioration of your psychological and mental capacities. Getting high is neither a form of higher consciousness nor does it help you achieve that state.

Tobacco is another no-go. You already know that smoking has detrimental effects on the lungs and on the brain. A major element in awakening your Kundalini is breathing and without your lungs to facilitate that action, you are doomed. Plus, smoking takes in dangerous toxins into your body, the very thing that we wish to avoid.

Ridding the body of toxins can also be done though body secretions. Run maintenance tasks on your vehicle through engaging in physical activities such as exercise. Sweat out the toxins from your body. But always remember not to overdo as any excess may lead to your body collapsing from the overworking. Moreover, don't shock your body into doing things it has never underwent before. If it's your first time to exercise, do not go all out and implement a training program containing an hour of cardio exercises, 2 hours on the treadmill, 100 crunches, and so on. You must gradually introduce your body to these activities and implement them slowly in order for the mind and body to adapt.

You can choose to run or bike for one hour a day to help the body be freed of the toxins. Put another resolution in your list which is to test and try your limits. If you can only bike for an hour, add another ten minutes the next time you do so. Use your mental power to push through your limitations. This will exercise your willpower and increase your concentration which you will need in awakening your Kundalini energy.

From time to time, you can have a full body massage to release the tension from your body. It would help in the better circulation of blood throughout your body and in opening up your chakra centers.

Other hormonal secretions must also leave the body before you undertake Kundalini awakening. If you are sexually tense and need a release, do it and don't robyourself of the opportunity. Restricting oneself would just prove to be detrimental since it would distract your mind from concentrating on the proper exercises when it's time.

Instead of relaxing and focusing on your breathing, you might end up fidgety and uncomfortable after the sexual repression.

Chapter 4: Umm and Ohms

In order to prepare and build your mind and body for Kundalini awakening, you must practice yoga and meditation. Meditating will familiarize you with the concentration and mental stability needed in spiritual exercises. You can start with simple meditation exercises such as emptying your mind and feeling your breathing. Another meditation exercise involves imagining a bright star whose light you will take in into your body.

If you immediately jump into doing the steps for Kundalini exercises, you might find it hard to focus without any prior experience.At first, you might find your thoughts careening around your mind like kids overdosed with candies. Any sound you will perceive can break your concentration and distract you. The first time trying to keep these thoughts in check would prove to be disastrous and exhausting. But, continuous engagement in trying to rein them in would make you more capable in the future. Meditation exercises will allow you to take control of your thoughts and their directions.

Do the meditation exercises as often as you can in order to train your mind. Your first ever Kundalini event may not prove as successful as intended because your mind haven't been trained enough to concentrate and focus.

Furthermore, practicing yoga will improve the connection between your mind and body. It refers to the joining together of the different consciousness in your body and mind. Yoga will allow you to realize your limitations and break through them. As you might have noticed in yoga exercises, there is an emphasis on how mental power can control the physical self. Through willpower and focus, you are able to execute physical postures and stances that you thought to be beyond your capabilities.

Sometimes, it's thinking of the words *no, can't,* and *impossible* that causes one's failures in any task. When your yoga instructor tells you to do a full lotus, negative thinking about the flexibility of your legs would make you not attempt to follow through. But if you train your mind to think *yes,* it's no longer mission impossible. Try to shift your perspective into a more positive one.

There are various yoga exercises that you can participate in as preparation for your Kundalini awakening which includes Hatha Yoga, Raja Yoga, and Bhakti Yoga. The steps that you can learn from the aforementioned forms of yoga can also be combined and used during your proper awakening. You can take elements from these yoga forms and prepare your mind and body through their combination.

Chapter 5: Rousing the Sleeping Serpent

Find a place or a spot you are comfortable in. It is important that you are at a place where your focus won't be easily broken or disrupted. Somewhere in nature is ideal. You can park yourself beside a pond, for example, or near a waterfall. However, if you do not have access to this kind of setting or don't have the time to reach one, you can choose a room that you can arrange to become more proper and suitable. Adjust the room's lighting and temperature. During the session, cellphones and other electronic devices must be turned off since they serve as distractions.

In lieu of the real deal, you can also decide to listen to some music of nature or just have silence as your company. Sounds of nature like that of flowing water and birds chirping could be ideal to stimulate the energy within you.

It is also important to start a session with the proper state of mind. If you are sick or troubled, it wouldn't be advised to follow through with the process. Pick a time wherein you don't have responsibilities and obligations to fulfill and answer to. Make sure that during the session, you would not be interrupted by your boss calling or a friend asking for a companion to the salon.

Prior to the session, you can also lower the stress level of your body by getting a full body massage in order to release the tension from your muscles.

Now, let's talk about the steps that you will need to master Kundalini awakening.

The first thing that you have to do is sit comfortably. Determine a position where you will not cramp your limbs or hurt any body part. Wear comfortable clothes, as well. Choose those which will not constrict your movements and your breathing. It would not do well to start awakening your Kundalini only to faint because your shirt is so tight that you can't breathe.

Inhale. Exhale. Breathe deeply. Regulate your breathing as rhythm is very important since it facilitates concentration.

Empty your mind of your daily worries. Stop thinking of the future and don't dwell in the past. Don't reminisce about your ex-loves and what you did at work earlier. Don't ponder on the trip that you have wanted to take for so many years now. Focus on the present and focus on your breathing.

As you breathe deeply, feel the air passing through your nose. Feel the oxygen passing through your nostrils and expanding your lungs with life.Inhale. Exhale. Feel the sensation of tranquility and peace embracing you. Feel the comfort embracing you as you continue breathing deeply. Relax your muscles. Feel the way your limbs are doing away with the tension. Feel your arms going loose. Be at ease with how your body feels.

Now, begin to focus your breathing at the base of your spine, the base chakra center. Feel your breathing. Fill your base chakra center with a pleasant sensation. Remember a time when you experienced a deep, pleasant sensation and fill the base of your spine with this feeling. Feel it opening and being filled with a pleasant feeling. Feel it opening and becoming filled with energy.

Continue to breathe deeply through your nose as you inhale and exhale. Allow the air to move into you, bringing life as it moves down into your lungs. Focus your breathing into your chest, at your heart. Feel it contracting as it pumps blood into your veins. Recall a memory when you felt a pleasant sensation at this center and bring that happy feeling into your heart. Think of a time when you were in love, when you felt elation and intense happiness. Feel your heart energizing, filling up with that wonderful sensation. Feel your heart and chest expanding with as they become full of the joyful sensation.

Bring your focus now in the middle of your neck. Breathe deeply. Inhale and exhale and concentrate on this area. Fill this chakra center with a pleasant sensation. Fill it up. Open it wider and wider and pour energy into it as you breathe deeply.

Continue to breathe deeply through your nose. Now concentrate on the next chakra center, on your third eye which is located on your forehead. Begin to breathe into this energy center. Feel the air energizing you and energizing this center. Feel your chakra energizing and think of a time when you felt a wonderful sensation in that area, something to make this energy center feel full. What about a beautiful memory. Bring the feeling from that moment into this moment. Open up this center and feel the clarity of thought, the absence of worries and clutters. Fill this center with positive sensation.

Bring your awareness now to your crown chakra located at the top of your head. Feel the energy moving through your body as you breathe deeply. Breathe and send the life the air gives you to your crown chakra. Feel it open and expand, becoming wider.

Bring your spine into a straight position. But do not forget to be comfortable. Relax your posture but straighten your spine. Feel your spine moving as it straightens. Feel every movement of your joints, vertebrae, as your spine becomes completely straight. Now, feel your energy center at the base of your spine. Breathe deeply into this energy center and feel it becoming open and active, widening and opening. Breathe deep.

Then breathe into the next energy center. Feel your chest expanding as the base of your spine is opening. Breathe deeply into both energy centers.

Breathe into the middle of your neck. Open this center and fill it with energy, with pleasant sensation. Breathe. Energize the three energy centers. Feel it brimming with sensation. Feel the wonderful sensation coursing throughout your body.

Focus now on your forehead. Make it active by pulling all the energy from the other centers into this center. Allow the energy to travel. Breathe deeply; let the energy flow from your nostrils into your lungs, into your spine and back up again into your chest, into your throat, and into your forehead.

Maintain your focus and continue to breathe deeply. Let the energy travel from the other energy centers into the energy center on your forehead. Fill it up with energy. Maintain the beautiful sensation of connection. Recall beautiful feelings and pour them into your energy centers.

Now, you are energizing every chakra center in your body. Feel the beautiful sensation all throughout your body. Maintain the pleasant sensations in these areas. Bring the energy from the base of the spine all the way up to your crown chakra.

Maintain the sense of depth and the sensations. Feel the connectedness within you. Continue to breathe deeply into these areas. When you are ready, begin to come back into your waking life with all these energy running through your body. Maintain your breathing. Open your eyes slowly and gradually come back to your wakeful existence.

Now, the energy is streaming through your body and the experience would last depending on how well you have executed the steps. The physical symptoms of the awakening may last up to 30 minutes and with repetition, you can lengthen this.

Alas! After only 30 minutes or even less, you have mastered Kundalini awakening. The degree to which your Kundalini may have arisen depends on your state of mind and your observance to the steps.

The movement of Kundalini, as it moves through the chakra centers, is felt in various physical manifestations. During the process, your body might tremble and an electric current might run along your spine as the energy in your chakra centers explode. There have been reports that during the flow of Kundalini upwards, sound like that of a flowing waterfall, tinkling ornaments, birds chirping, may be internally perceived and heard. Your mouth may also fill with saliva. The symptoms may also differ across situations. In one session, you may feel your head getting heady and feel bright lights behind your eyes but in another session may hear sounds and feel sexual tension.

The experience will not be identical on every individual. Don't worry if what you go through differs from what you've heard since it is affected by your specific situation.

Remember to relax your focus. Don't force it. As you focus the energy up from the chakra centers in the lower parts of your body up towards your crown chakra center, you allow the energy to move on its own.

Moreover, don't think that the steps are too ridiculous to perform. You might wonder why and how you could focus your breathing into energy centers where air doesn't normally flow into. But it's actually effective to think of your breathing as a way of moving your energy around. When you focus your breathing in a specific chakra center, the energy flows to that area.

Chapter 6: It's Complicated

Now that you are aware of the steps you need to take to master Kundalini, take the first steps towards your spiritual journey. However, you must heed some warnings regarding this mystical adventure. In every endeavor, there are always risks when they're not done with prior knowledge and preparation.

In the case of Kundalini, there is such a thing as premature awakening. Not everyone is fit to have their energy awakened. Let's take physical exercise as an example. If you are like the majority of people who have hated PE classes when they were required during high school and college, you probably forsake any kind of task that puts demands you to strenuously move. But let's say that a circumstance has come up and it expects you to exercise through jumping over ropes 100 times in a minute. Can you do it? Maybe you have arthritis or maybe your body is not just strong enough for this kind of physical torture. The answer, then, is *No*. So, should you push it? Again, *No!* If you will, you would probably end up face first on the floor. This logic also applies to Kundalini awakening. A balanced and strong mind coupled with a balanced personality and body is needed as raising Kundalini demands a great deal of energy and willpower.

When either the mind or body is unprepared, it can be overwhelmed and this would lead to complications. The experience felt when this is the case is called *Kundalini syndrome.*

One's nervous system could be overloaded. In this situation, you'll end up in a ward, dressed in white and screaming "I'm not crazy" to the staff, because of a psychotic break. An unprepared person could also suffer disassociation from reality as a result of hasty proceedings. You might end up believing you're in Hogwarts even when you are obviously not.To add, severe anxiety wherein you will worry over the simplest of things could render you incapable of performing daily activities. Additionally, there were reports of disorientations and physical complications like sexual dysfunctions and gastrointestinal disorders (Kundalini Complications, ND). Insomnia and involuntary movements could also result from premature awakening.

These complications from premature arousal is explained to be consequences of one's Kundalini energy encountering barriers as it progresses from the base of your spine to the top of your head. These barriers could be in the form of toxins that one didn't eradicate from the body or even thoughts that proved to be disruptive to the flow of energy.

Going through the awakening while your mental state is so troubled that no meditation can empty it is a no-no. Aggression, violence, and other negative dispositions could also be detrimental. Negative emotions will always be discouraged because in an effort that involves the spirit, malevolent thoughts and feelings are not welcome.

So remember to not take the immediate plunge towards Kundalini arousal. Remember the tips – understand Kundalini, purify your body of the toxins, and meditate.They are recommended for a valid reason which is to ready your body and mind.

Conclusion

Thank you again for downloading this book!

I hope this book was able to help you to become more familiar with what Kundalini is. You might just have heard of Kundalini from your neighbor and thought it as another Indian fad. But at this point, you know that it is more than that as it is a long-term goal that requires dedication, hard work, and faith. You are now equipped with the knowledge regarding this delicate spiritual journey. I hope this book was also able to teach you what you need to do before you engage in rousing your inner serpent and guide you with the steps in doing so. Take note of the importance of adequate knowledge, proper meditation, and a balanced mind and body.

The next step is to take heed of the tips and warnings that come with triggering your spiritual energy. You are now armed with guiding words into taking that step towards a higher state of consciousness and enlightenment.

Remember that this spiritual path must not be taken out of boredom or simple curiosity. It takes commitment and discipline in order to stick to the principles of Kundalini.

Finally, if you enjoyed this book, please take the time to share your thoughts and post a review on Amazon. It'd be greatly appreciated!

Thank you and good luck!

Made in the USA
Columbia, SC
28 April 2022

59602449R00067